Anchors of Support

Building a Legacy of Stability for Families Navigating Mental Illness

Dr. Cindy H. Carr, D.Min. MACL
The Anchored Series

This book is published by **CHC Connect**.

All views and opinions expressed in this work are those of the author. Any errors or omissions are unintentional.

Printed in the United States of America
First Edition, 2026

ISBN: 978-1-971192-20-8

For permissions or inquiries, contact:
Cindy H. Carr
cindyhcarr@outlook.com
www.cindyhcarr.com

Acknowledgements

To my husband, Walter W. ("Dubby") Carr III— thank you for building this legacy of stability and love with me. You have walked beside me through seasons of joy and seasons of strain, and you have taught me what steady partnership looks like when life is complicated. Our story has never been perfect, but it has been faithful, and I am grateful for the way you keep choosing "us."

I also want to acknowledge the many teachers, mentors, clinicians, and faith leaders whose wisdom has shaped the way I serve families. Much of what is most helpful in this book has been learned in holy places—through prayer, through Scripture, through the quiet work of counseling rooms, and through the courageous families who have trusted me with their stories.

Finally, to every caregiver reading these pages: thank you. Your love is often unseen, your labor often misunderstood, and your strength often stretched thin. My prayer is that this book gives you language, structure, and hope—so you can build support that lasts and protect what is sacred in your home.

How to Use This Book

You do not have to read this book straight through. You can read it in whatever way serves your season.

Here are three simple options:

• Quick Start (First Week): Read Chapters 1–4, then complete Tool #1 (Crisis Readiness Sheet) and Tool #24 (Family Living Plan).

• Build the Team (Next Month): Read one chapter per week and add tools as you need them. Focus on building your Anchors of Support and clarifying boundaries with bridges.

• Full Foundation (Ongoing): Read the entire book, then revisit chapters and tools anytime life changes, symptoms shift, or capacity changes.

At the end of each chapter you'll find: a Legacy Takeaway, a Next Step, a toolkit reference, and a first-person prayer you can pray directly to God.

A Note to the Reader

If mental illness has touched your home, you already know this is not a simple journey. Some days feel calm and ordinary. Other days feel like you're holding the whole system together with your bare hands.

This book was written to give you a structure that can hold—without asking you to become a clinician, and without reducing your loved one to a diagnosis. My goal is to help you build a collaborative approach to care: a sustainable plan that can be renegotiated as life changes, and a home environment where connection and purpose remain non-negotiable.

You'll find practical tools in the Toolkit Appendix so the chapters can stay clean and conversational. Use the tools in whatever order fits your family. If you only start with two, start with the Crisis Readiness Sheet and the Family Living Plan.

We are building one main thing throughout this book: a legacy of stability.

Table of Contents

Chapter 1
The Main Thing: A Legacy of Stability Is Never Built Alone

Families often measure success by whether life feels calm. Calm matters. Peace matters. But when mental illness is involved, calm cannot be the only measure, because calm is not always available on demand. Some seasons will be steady, and other seasons will be stormy. The question becomes: what holds the family when the storm comes?

This is where a different goal changes everything. Instead of aiming for a perfect season, families can aim for a legacy: a long story shaped by safety, dignity, connection, and purpose. A legacy is built over time. It accounts for setbacks without calling them failure. It allows the family to keep moving forward even when symptoms return, plans need adjusting, or grief resurfaces.

A legacy of stability is never built alone. Yet families often try. Many people quietly believe, "If I am strong enough, calm enough, wise enough, spiritual enough, I can hold this." But strength without support turns into strain. Strain turns into resentment. Resentment turns into distance. And distance is the opposite of what a struggling person and a struggling family needs.

When families are in "hero mode," a few patterns tend to show up. One person becomes the primary stabilizer and begins to disappear as a person. Children begin to monitor adult emotions, becoming anxious or hyper-responsible. The home becomes reactive, always responding, rarely restoring. The family starts to confuse love with self-erasure.

If any of that sounds familiar, please hear this with kindness: your exhaustion is not evidence that you are failing. It may be evidence that you are carrying more than one household was ever meant to carry.

In the pages ahead, you will learn practical skills: how to de-escalate, how to set boundaries that protect dignity, how to rebuild rhythm, how to create a crisis plan, how to teach children honor and safety at the same time. But the first and most important decision is not a skill. It is a shift in posture: you will stop trying to do this alone.

For many families, this shift begins with one question: Who is holding this with us? Not who is judging us. Not who is offering opinions from the outside. Who is truly holding the rope with you, steadily, kindly, and in the right role?

That question matters because mental illness often creates confusion about responsibility. Families can start to believe they are responsible for outcomes they cannot control. They can start to believe that if the person does not improve, it means they did not love enough, pray enough, or do enough. That weight is crushing, and it is not yours to carry alone. Love is not measured by whether you can fix what you did not cause.

This book will repeatedly return you to a simple, freeing truth: stability is a team outcome. When families build the right kind of support, they can stop living in cycles of panic and repair. They can begin to respond with wisdom instead of fear. They can protect the home without abandoning the person. And they can define healing in a way that allows wholeness to be possible, even when limitations remain.

Legacy Takeaway

The goal is not to become the hero. The goal is to build a team. A legacy of stability is built through shared support that protects safety, dignity, connection, and purpose.

Next Step

Choose one trusted person and share one truthful sentence this week: "We're carrying more than we can manage alone, and we're building support." If you do not have that person yet, your next step is to identify where your support can begin (clinical, medical, community, or home team).

Toolkit link:

Tool #2 — Anchors of Support Map.

Closing Prayer

God, give me courage to step out of isolation and into shared support. Help me release the belief that I have to carry this alone. Teach me to build stability with wisdom and grace, and to protect what is sacred in our home: safety, dignity, connection, and purpose. Strengthen me for today, and guide us one step at a time. Amen.

Chapter 2
The Four Anchors of Support: Building a Team That Holds

Most families do not set out to carry mental illness alone. It happens gradually. A loved one struggles, the family responds, and the responding becomes the new normal. You adjust your schedules. You watch your words. You manage moods. You learn which topics set off conflict and which routines calm things down. Over time, you can become so focused on keeping the day afloat that you forget a simple truth: one household was never designed to be the whole system.

When a family tries to become everything, therapist, prescriber, pastor, crisis team, and constant emotional regulator, the home begins to run on strain instead of strength. And strain changes the atmosphere. Children feel it. Couples feel it. The person who is unwell feels it too, even when they cannot name it. This is one reason I talk about support in a different way. We do not just need "help." We need a structure that holds. We need anchors.

I call this framework The Four Anchors of Support because it gives families language for what they already sense: stability requires more than love and good intentions. Anchors do not erase storms. Anchors hold you steady when the storm comes. They keep the home from drifting into chaos and the caregiver from collapsing under expectations no human can carry alone.

The anchors are simple to name, but powerful to live out: a Clinical Anchor, a Medical Anchor, a Community Anchor, and a Home Team Anchor. Most families already have one or two of these in place. The trouble begins when an anchor is missing, or when one anchor is forced to carry the weight of all four. In those seasons, even strong families start to feel like they are failing, when what is really happening is that the structure is incomplete.

The Clinical Anchor is the place where skills are built. A therapist or counselor helps a person learn how to regulate emotions, name patterns, rebuild thinking habits, repair relationships, and recover from trauma that still lives in the nervous system. Clinical care is not just "talking." Done well, it becomes a training ground for stability, because insight without skills rarely changes daily life. Families often find relief when they stop asking, "Why are they like this?" and start asking, "What skills can we build, and what supports do we need while they grow?"

The Medical Anchor recognizes a truth many families learn the hard way: the brain is an organ. When the brain is unhealthy or injured, it can affect mood, perception, impulse control, sleep, motivation, and even the ability to connect. A prescriber, psychiatrist, or physician helps evaluate what is happening biologically and neurologically and considers treatment options that may include medication, sleep support, nutrition, and other medical interventions. Medication is not a moral failure. It is one tool among many, sometimes life-saving, sometimes temporary, sometimes part of long-term management. The point is not to win a debate about medication. The point is to build stability with wisdom and humility.

The Community Anchor is where belonging lives. This may be a faith community, a recovery community, a support group, or a circle of trusted people who can hold the family with practical care and steady compassion. Community is not meant to replace clinicians. Community cannot diagnose, prescribe, or carry legal responsibility for treatment. But community can do something sacred that professionals cannot: it can offer consistent belonging. It can reduce shame. It can show up with meals, rides, prayer, texts, childcare, and presence. When community stays in its lane, it becomes one of the strongest stabilizers a family can have.

The Home Team Anchor is the daily environment. It is the family, the friends, and the close support people who learn how to respond without shame, how to set boundaries that protect dignity, and how to protect children without making them responsible for adult burdens. Home Team support includes routines, calm communication, repair after conflict, and practical plans for hard days. It includes learning how to de-escalate, when to step back, and when to call for help. It is the anchor that keeps the home from becoming a revolving door of crisis and exhaustion.

Here is the quiet truth that changes everything: you do not have to be all four anchors. You only have to build them. And building them is a process. Some families begin with clinical care. Some begin with medical stability. Some begin by finally letting community in. Some begin by strengthening the home team so children can breathe again. Wherever you begin, the goal is the same: shared support that is clear, consistent, and sustainable.

As you read this book, you will keep returning to one simple question: Which anchor is strongest right now, and which anchor is most at risk? If you can answer that honestly, you will almost always know your next faithful step. Not your next perfect step, your next faithful one. The kind that creates stability over time.

And one more word of encouragement: you are not behind. You are not late to the work. Many families do not learn these anchors until they are already exhausted. If that is you, let this framework bring you relief, not pressure. We are not building a flawless system. We are building a structure that holds love in place when life gets hard.

Legacy Takeaway

Stability is a team outcome. When the Four Anchors of Support are active and shared, love becomes sustainable and the home becomes steadier, even in complicated stories.

Next Step

Do an honest Anchor Check: Which anchor is currently carrying the most weight in your family, clinical, medical, community, or home team? Then choose one small step to strengthen the weakest or missing anchor this week.

Toolkit link:

Tool #3 — Weekly Anchor Check (Reset).

Closing Prayer

God, give me wisdom to build shared support with humility and courage. Show me which anchor is weak or missing, and guide me toward the right help in the right lane. Strengthen our home team with grace, surround us with community, and help us use clinical and medical care wisely. Teach me to measure faithfulness by steady love, not by carrying what was never mine to carry alone. Amen.

Chapter 3
The Battery Starts Low: Why "Just Try Harder" Doesn't Work

One of the most common misunderstandings families carry is this: they assume the person who is struggling has the same internal capacity they do. So when the person can't follow through, can't stay regulated, can't show up, can't "snap out of it," the family starts to interpret the struggle as choice, laziness, defiance, or lack of faith. That interpretation is not only inaccurate, it quietly poisons the relationship.

I use a simple image to explain what is happening: the battery. Many people wake up with a battery that is more or less charged. They may be tired, stressed, or distracted, but they can move through the day, complete basic tasks, and recover after hard moments. For many people living with mental illness, the battery starts low before the day even begins. They are not choosing to be depleted. Their nervous system is already working overtime.

When your battery starts low, everything costs more. A text message can feel like a mountain. A phone call can feel like danger. A crowded store can feel like a fire alarm. A normal conflict can flood the body with panic. Even good things, holidays, family gatherings, celebrations, can drain a low battery faster than anyone expects. Families often say, "But nothing even happened today." And the truth may be: nothing happened externally. But internally, the body has been fighting for stability all day long.

This is why "just try harder" fails. It assumes that willpower is the problem. It assumes the person has full access to regulation, motivation, and reasoning at the very moment those systems may be impaired. When the brain is under stress, the rational center can go offline. People can lose access to skills they actually do have. They can say things they don't mean. They can shut down. They can escalate. And afterward, shame floods in because they don't understand why they couldn't do what seems simple to everyone else.

Families also start to fail when they define success as a symptom-free life. If symptom erasure is the only definition of healing, then every flare-up feels like failure. But symptoms often come in waves. Some conditions are episodic. Some are chronic. Some improve over time with treatment and rhythm. Some remain stubborn. This is why we define success differently in this book. We define progress by stability markers: safety increasing, connection protected, rhythm returning, support shared, and purpose preserved.

Understanding the battery helps families make a crucial shift: you stop arguing about character and start building support. You stop saying, "You should be able to do this," and start asking, "What would make this possible?" Sometimes the answer is clinical skill-building. Sometimes it is medical support. Sometimes it is sleep and rhythm. Sometimes it is boundaries that protect overstimulation. Sometimes it is community. Often it is a combination. The question is not, "Who is wrong?" The question is, "What does our system need?"

This is also where caregivers need compassion for themselves. When you live beside a low-battery reality, you can begin to drain too. You may become hyper-alert, scanning the room for mood shifts and tension. You may start walking on eggshells. You may start overfunctioning, doing too much because you're afraid what will happen if you don't. Over time, your battery starts low as well. Then the whole home is running on depletion.

One of the kindest things you can do for a struggling person is to stop shaming what they cannot control and start helping them build what they can. That does not mean you tolerate harm. It means you learn how to set boundaries that protect dignity, how to de-escalate when the nervous system is flooded, and how to strengthen the Anchors of Support so no one person is carrying the whole weight.

If you are reading this and thinking, "But my person uses the illness as an excuse," you are not alone. Some people do avoid responsibility. Some do manipulate. Some do refuse help. This book will not ask you to pretend that does not exist. What it will do is help you separate illness from choices, and help you respond in a way that is both compassionate and wise. You can honor a person's dignity and still require safe behavior. You can believe the struggle is real and still insist on support, treatment, and boundaries.

So let's make this practical. When your loved one is low-battery, your goal is not to win an argument. Your goal is to reduce overload, protect connection, and choose the next step that strengthens stability. That is how families endure. That is how a legacy of stability is built, one steady day at a time.

Legacy Takeaway

A low battery changes what is possible. When families stop shaming depletion and start building support, stability becomes more attainable and connection stays protected.

Next Step

Notice one moment this week when you are tempted to say, "Just try harder." Replace it with one stabilizing question: "What would make this doable right now?" Then choose one small adjustment, sleep, rhythm, reduced stimulation, a clinical skill, a medical check-in, or added community support, that strengthens the weakest anchor.

Toolkit link:

Tool #11 — Trigger + Pattern Tracker (Experience-Based).

Closing Prayer

God, give me wisdom to see what is happening beneath the behavior. Help me respond with compassion and truth, without shame, without fear, and without denial. Teach me to build stability through shared support, steady rhythm, and wise boundaries. Strengthen my heart when the battery is low, and help our home stay anchored in safety, dignity, connection, and purpose. Amen. [1][4]

Chapter 4
Sleep, Rhythm, and Grace: Rest as a Stabilizing Gift

If you want to stabilize a home, start with the body. That may sound too simple for something as complex as mental illness, but it is one of the most compassionate places to begin. When sleep is broken, everything gets harder: mood regulation, impulse control, memory, motivation, patience, and connection. When sleep improves, the whole system gains a little more margin. And margin is often the difference between a hard day and a crisis.

Many families treat sleep like a reward: "When you behave, you can rest." Or they treat sleep like a moral issue: "If you really wanted to, you would go to bed." But sleep is not a character trait. It is a biological rhythm. God wired our bodies with internal timing, circadian rhythms that regulate sleep and wake cycles, hunger patterns, hormone release, alertness, and recovery. When we honor those rhythms, rest comes more easily. When we fight them, everyone suffers.

I've learned this personally. I'm an early-to-bed, early-to-rise person. My mind begins to wind down in the evening, and some of my clearest thinking comes in the quiet hours before dawn. My husband is wired differently. His mind often wakes up at night, and he naturally sleeps later. For years, I assumed one of us needed to "fix" it. Now I see it as one of the ways God designed us differently. The goal was never to force sameness. The goal was to build a rhythm that respected both of us and protected the home.

That same truth matters even more when mental illness is in the story. Sleep disruption can mimic or intensify symptoms. A person who is sleep-deprived may appear more anxious, more irritable, more impulsive, more depressed, or more dysregulated. For some, sleep loss can trigger severe destabilization. For others, sleep becomes a battleground because the nervous system does not feel safe enough to rest. Families can end up arguing about bedtime when what they are really dealing with is biology, trauma, and chronic stress.

So how do we approach sleep with both structure and grace? We start with one principle: stability grows when rhythms are predictable. Predictable does not mean perfect. It means repeatable. It means the home has cues that tell the body, "You are safe. You can downshift. You can recover."

Here are a few practical guardrails that help most families, without turning bedtime into a power struggle. First, anchor the wake-up time. Many people try to fix sleep by focusing only on bedtime. But wake-up time sets the rhythm of the day. When wake-up times are wildly inconsistent, the body struggles to find its natural timing. If you can anchor wake-up time within a reasonable window, sleep often begins to stabilize over time.

Second, build a wind-down window. Most people cannot go from screens, stress, and stimulation straight into deep sleep. A wind-down window is a gentle transition. Lights lower. Noise softens. Screens go quiet. The body receives repeated cues: the day is ending. This window might be twenty minutes or ninety minutes depending on the person, but it should be consistent enough that the brain learns the pattern.

Third, reduce shame. Families often shame sleep patterns because they feel out of control: "You're lazy." "You're irresponsible." "You're wasting the day." Shame does not restore rhythm. Shame increases stress, and stress interrupts sleep. If you need boundaries around sleep because the home must function, work schedules, school schedules, responsibilities, that is real. But boundaries can be held with dignity: "Our home needs a rhythm. Let's build a plan we can live with."

Fourth, remember that sleep is not one-size-fits-all. Some people are sunrise risers. Some are night thinkers. Many adolescents experience biological shifts that make them sleepy later and wake later. Some adults carry a nervous system that doesn't settle until the house is quiet. The goal is not to force everyone into the same clock. The goal is to build enough rhythm that the body can recover and the home can function.

And here is the grace piece: sometimes sleep won't cooperate quickly. Medication changes, trauma triggers, grief, mania, anxiety spirals, pain, or life disruption can all break sleep. In those seasons, sleep becomes part of the care plan, not a behavior plan. That means you strengthen the medical and clinical anchors, you protect rhythm where you can, you reduce stimulation, and you let the home team support the person without turning sleep into a shame cycle.

Parents and caregivers, if bedtime has become a battlefield, take heart. You are not failing. You are navigating biology, development, and the individuality of a person God designed with complexity. Lead with structure and grace, not fear and frustration. Rest is not surrender. Rest is part of how the brain heals and how the body regains stability.

In the chapters ahead, we will talk about regulation, de-escalation, and boundaries. But I want you to remember this: when sleep improves, everything else is easier to practice. Sleep doesn't solve everything, but it gives the family a fighting chance. And sometimes, that is exactly what you need to keep building a legacy of stability.

Legacy Takeaway

Rhythm is a form of care. When a home honors sleep with structure and grace, the nervous system gains margin, and margin makes stability more attainable.

Next Step

Choose one rhythm reset that is realistic for your home this week: (1) anchor wake-up time within a consistent window, (2) create a 30–60 minute wind-down routine, or (3) reduce one major sleep disruptor (late screens, caffeine timing, overstimulation). Keep it small and repeatable.

Toolkit link:

Tool #6 — Sleep + Rhythm Reset (7 Days, Grace-Based).

Closing Prayer

God, teach me to lead our home with rhythm and grace. Help me build rest without shame and structure without power struggles. Give us wisdom to honor how You wired our bodies, courage to set healthy guardrails, and compassion in seasons when sleep is hard. Let rest become a stabilizing gift in our home, and strengthen the support we need for long-term endurance. Amen. [3][4]

Chapter 5
Connection and Purpose:
The Non-Negotiables

When mental illness enters a family story, it can quietly rewrite the family's priorities. Without meaning to, the home begins to revolve around symptoms: keeping someone calm, preventing a blow-up, managing the next appointment, recovering from the last crisis. Families can become so focused on stopping the storm that they lose sight of what the storm is threatening most, connection and purpose.

I want to say this plainly: connection and purpose are not "nice extras." For a person living with mental illness, connection is stabilizing. Purpose is stabilizing. They are among the most protective factors we have. And that is why they are non-negotiable. Even when behavior is hard. Even when the family is tired. Even when boundaries are needed. We protect connection and purpose because they are often the very bridge that keeps someone from drifting into deeper isolation, shame, and despair.

This can feel complicated, especially when other vulnerable adults are affected by behaviors that are a result of mental illness. A spouse gets worn down. Siblings get anxious. Grandparents get overwhelmed.

Caregivers get depleted. So let me be clear about what I mean by connection. Connection does not mean constant access. Connection does not mean unlimited closeness. Connection means the person is not made "junk" in the family story. It means we keep dignity intact while we protect safety.

Sometimes protecting connection requires rotating the lead caregiver. Many families burn out because one responsible person becomes the permanent stabilizer, and everyone else assumes they can keep going. But capacity is real. Some people are wired with a larger capacity, and others have a smaller one. Some seasons expand capacity, and other seasons shrink it. Wisdom is knowing the difference, and adjusting without shame.

Rotating leadership can be as simple as this: one caregiver handles appointments and medication communication for a season, another handles school coordination and routines, another becomes the person who takes the evening shift when symptoms are most intense. Rotating the lead does not mean rotating love. It means protecting the home team so your support is sustainable. The goal is not a superhuman caregiver. The goal is a steady family.

Connection also requires a new understanding of boundaries. In the last chapter we talked about guardrails that protect safety and dignity. Here's the connection piece: boundaries should never be designed to break relationship, value, or purpose. If a boundary is needed, it should come with a bridge. A bridge can be a next step: "We can talk when we're calm." "I will meet you at your appointment." "I'm not able to do that, but I can do this." A boundary without a bridge often feels like rejection, and rejection is gasoline on the fire for many people who already feel ashamed or afraid.

Purpose is the other stabilizer families often lose. When a person is unwell, life can shrink down to survival: medication, symptoms, sleep, conflict, recovery. But human beings are not built to live without meaning. Purpose does not have to be big or public. Purpose can be small and consistent: a hobby, a creative outlet, a job task, a volunteer role, a spiritual practice, a daily responsibility that fits the person's capacity. Purpose says, "You still matter here." It says, "You still have something to offer."

This is where families can make a powerful shift. Instead of asking only, "How do we stop the behavior?" you also ask, "How do we protect connection and purpose while we manage the behavior?" That question keeps the home from becoming only a crisis center. It keeps the family from becoming only a treatment plan. It keeps the person from becoming only a diagnosis.

And let's talk about children, because this is one of the tender places where connection and purpose matter most. A parent with mental illness is still valuable to a child, even if they cannot be the primary caregiver. Children need truth, and children need honor. We can teach both at the same time. We can say, "Your parent loves you. Your parent is sick right now. The sickness affects choices and emotions. Our job is to keep you safe and loved. You are not responsible for the illness." We can protect children without teaching contempt.

When families do this well, children grow up with something priceless: they learn that love can be honest. They learn that dignity doesn't disappear when someone is unwell. They learn that boundaries can exist without hatred. They learn that family can be complicated and still be sacred.

If you're wondering how to live this out when the behavior is intense, remember the Four Anchors. Connection and purpose become much easier to protect when the support is shared. Clinical care can help build relational skills. Medical care can reduce destabilizing symptoms. Community can provide belonging. The home team can create rhythm and guardrails. Together, the anchors protect the non-negotiables.

So here is the question I want you to carry forward: what would it look like to protect connection and purpose in your home this week, without denying reality? You don't have to solve the whole story today. You simply have to keep the main thing the main thing. Connection. Purpose. Dignity. Safety. And a plan that can be renegotiated as life changes.

Legacy Takeaway

Connection and purpose stabilize the mind and protect the family story. Even when boundaries are needed, dignity and relationship must remain intact.

Next Step

Choose one connection move and one purpose move for this week. Connection move: a short, calm check-in, a walk, a shared meal, or a kind text that does not try to fix. Purpose move: one small role or meaningful activity that fits current capacity. Keep both simple and repeatable.

Toolkit link:

Tool #14 — Connection + Purpose Plan (Capacity-Based).

Closing Prayer

God, help me protect connection and purpose in our home, even when the road is hard. Give me wisdom to set boundaries with bridges, courage to tell the truth with dignity, and humility to share the load with others. Show me how to honor each person's value, especially when someone is unwell, and help us build a steady, sustainable plan that can grow and change with each season. Amen.

Chapter 6
Shared Care: Keeping Everyone in Their Lane

By now, you can probably feel the theme of this book: no one heals alone, and no family can carry mental illness well without shared support. That sounds simple, but the moment real life hits, an outburst, a missed appointment, a medication change, a relapse, a school problem, a crisis call, families often collapse back into the same pattern: the responsible person tries to do everything.

This chapter is here to stop that cycle. Not by giving you more to do, but by helping you keep everyone in their lane. Because when roles get blurry, families burn out. And when families burn out, stability becomes harder for everyone, including the person who is struggling.

Let's name the common role confusion. A spouse becomes the therapist. A parent becomes the prescriber. A pastor becomes a crisis clinician. A friend becomes a case manager. A child becomes an emotional support partner. A church becomes the only source of care. None of those roles are sustainable. And none of them are what God designed a healthy support system to be.

This is why the Four Anchors of Support matter so much. They do not just give you "help." They give you structure. And structure is what keeps love from becoming exhaustion.

Here is what it looks like when the lanes are clear.

The Clinical Anchor helps build skills. The clinician's role is to help a person understand patterns, process trauma, build emotional regulation, learn communication tools, and practice new ways of responding under stress. Clinical care also helps families learn what is realistic, what is unsafe, and what needs a plan. The clinician is not there to be your family referee. The clinician is there to build capacity and stability over time.

The Medical Anchor addresses brain-and-body realities. The medical role is to evaluate symptoms, consider diagnosis, manage medication when appropriate, and look for biological contributors like sleep disruption, substance interactions, hormone shifts, nutritional deficiencies, neurological conditions, or other medical factors that can imitate or intensify mental health symptoms. The medical role is not to provide long-term talk therapy. It is to bring medical wisdom to the care plan.

The Community Anchor provides belonging. Faith communities and other support communities can surround families with compassion, prayer, meals, rides, childcare, accountability, and a sense of purpose. Community is powerful because it reduces shame and isolation. But community must stay in its lane. Community does not diagnose. Community does not prescribe. Community does not replace crisis services. Community does not become the only support while clinical and medical needs go untreated. When community stays in its lane, it becomes one of the greatest gifts a family can receive.

The Home Team Anchor is the daily environment, the people who live close enough to the story that they feel the impact. The home team's role is to protect safety and dignity, build rhythm, hold boundaries, practice repair, and follow the plan. The home team is not responsible for curing the illness. The home team is responsible for creating a stable, respectful environment where healing work can actually take root.

Now here is the part that changes everything: you do not strengthen your system by asking one anchor to do another anchor's job. You strengthen your system by building communication between the anchors, so the care plan is coordinated and sustainable.

This is what I mean by collaborative care. Collaborative care is not complicated. It is simply shared responsibility with clear roles. It is the family saying, "We are not trying to manage this as a dominant. We are building a community of support." It is the caregiver learning the difference between support and control. It is the clinician and prescriber doing their work while the home team builds rhythm and boundaries. It is the community offering belonging without trying to replace professional care.

Families often ask, "But how do we actually coordinate this without turning our lives into a full-time job?" Start small. You do not need a formal team meeting to begin. You need one clear plan that everyone can point to. You need one or two agreed-upon communication habits. And you need permission to stop carrying what isn't yours.

Here are three practical ways to keep lanes clear.

First, name the role out loud. When you feel yourself becoming the therapist, the prescriber, or the crisis team, pause and say, "That is not my lane." Then ask, "Which anchor does this belong to?" The simple act of naming the lane reduces panic and helps you choose the right next step.

Second, build a short list of "who to call for what." In a stable season, create a small contact list: clinician, prescriber, crisis support options, trusted community supports, and home team roles. In a crisis season, your brain will not have the capacity to invent a plan. A plan needs to already exist.

Third, protect the children from role drift. Children should never be the anchor for adult stability. They should not be the confidant, the mediator, the emotional support spouse, or the crisis manager. Children can love a struggling parent. Children can be honest about feelings. But children must remain children. This is one of the strongest ways you build a legacy of stability.

If you are thinking, "This sounds good, but my person refuses help," I understand. Some families are trying to build anchors while the person resists. The truth is: you can still strengthen the home team, increase community support, and clarify boundaries even if the person is not fully participating yet. You can still stop role confusion. You can still protect children. You can still build a structure that holds. Sometimes, the system getting healthier is what makes it possible for the struggling person to accept help later.

And if you are the one who has been carrying everything, I want you to hear a gentle word: stepping back into your lane is not abandonment. It is wisdom. It is stewardship. It is love that lasts. You are not quitting. You are building something sustainable.

So as we move into the next section of the book, keep this in front of you: your goal is not to do more. Your goal is to do what is yours to do, and to build the anchors that make stability a shared outcome. That is how families endure. That is how connection stays protected. That is how a legacy is built.

Legacy Takeaway

When everyone stays in their lane, care becomes sustainable. Collaborative support protects the home, preserves dignity, and keeps children from carrying adult burdens.

Next Step

Create a one-page "Who Does What" plan: list your Clinical Anchor, Medical Anchor, Community Anchor, and Home Team roles. Write one sentence under each: what they do, and what they do not do. Keep it simple and accessible.

Toolkit link:

Tool #1 — Anchors of Support Map + Tool #4 — Collaborative Care Contact List.

Closing Prayer

God, give me humility to stay in my lane and courage to ask for shared support. Help me release what I was never meant to carry alone. Teach our family to build collaborative care with clear roles, wise boundaries, and steady love. Protect our children from adult burdens, and strengthen every anchor so our home can remain safe, dignified, connected, and purposeful. Amen.

Chapter 7
Honoring a Parent Who Is Unwell: Protecting Kids Without Making Anyone "Junk"

Some of the deepest pain in families affected by mental illness is not only what happens to the person who is struggling. It is what happens to the children who love them. Children can carry confusion, fear, loyalty conflicts, grief, anger, and shame, sometimes all in the same week. And if the adults don't give children a dignifying framework, children will invent one. They will often assume the worst about themselves.

This is why I say this plainly: a parent with mental illness is still valuable to a child, even if they cannot be the primary caregiver. Mental illness may reduce a parent's capacity. It may limit what is safe. It may change the rhythm of involvement. But it does not erase worth. It does not erase parenthood. And it should not erase honor.

Now, when I use the word honor, I'm not talking about pretending everything is fine. I'm not talking about sending children into unsafe situations. I'm not talking about telling children to tolerate harm. Honor is not denial. Honor is dignity. Honor is the refusal to make someone "junk" in the family story, even when we must set strong boundaries.

Families often swing to extremes. One extreme is secrecy: we don't talk about it, we don't name it, we just hope it goes away. The other extreme is contempt: we label the unwell parent as selfish, crazy, useless, or dangerous, and children absorb that tone like oxygen. Both extremes harm a child's heart. Secrecy creates confusion. Contempt creates hatred and identity wounds, because half of the child comes from that parent.

The healthier way is truth with tenderness. We tell children what is true in age-appropriate language. We name the illness without making it the person's identity. We explain behavior without excusing harm. We protect children without shaming the parent. And we keep the child out of adult emotional responsibility.

This can sound like simple sentences. "Your mom loves you, and she is sick right now." "Your dad's brain is struggling, and it affects his moods." "The sickness can make it hard for your parent to be consistent." "You did not cause this." "You cannot fix it." "You are safe, and the adults are building a plan." Those sentences become a stabilizing script when life feels unpredictable.

Children also need clarity about responsibility. When a parent is unwell, children often feel like they must become the peacekeeper, the caretaker, the translator, or the emotional support spouse. That role drift is incredibly common, and it is damaging. It can create anxiety, perfectionism, hypervigilance, and later relational patterns where the child thinks love equals rescuing.

So we protect children by putting adults back in adult roles. If a child is mediating conflict between parents, we stop it. If a child is managing medication reminders, we stop it. If a child is taking the emotional temperature of the home and shaping themselves around it, we intervene. We don't do that by scolding the child. We do it by building a stronger home team and a clearer plan.

This is also where boundaries matter. Sometimes a parent cannot be the primary caregiver. Sometimes visitation must be supervised. Sometimes contact must be limited. Sometimes the home must be structured around safety needs. Those decisions can carry intense guilt for families. But if safety requires a boundary, the boundary is not an attack on the parent's worth. It is protection of what is sacred: the child's nervous system, the child's development, and the child's experience of stability.

At the same time, we keep a bridge whenever possible. A boundary without a bridge often communicates rejection. A bridge can be a supervised visit, a scheduled call, a letter, a shared activity, or a trusted adult present. A bridge can also be the way we speak about the parent when the parent is not in the room. Children should not have to choose love for one parent by hating the other.

I've seen families do this well even in heartbreaking circumstances. A grandparent becomes the day-to-day caregiver while a parent receives treatment. A co-parent steps into primary structure while the other parent stabilizes. A child lives with one household while keeping meaningful, safe connection with the other. These are not perfect stories. They are adaptive stories. And they can still be sacred.

This chapter also matters for blended families, kinship care, and guardianship situations, because the adult raising the child may not be the child's biological parent. In those homes, honor becomes even more important. Children benefit from learning: "My story can be complicated, and I am still whole." They benefit from knowing that love can show up in many forms without shaming the people who could not carry what they wished they could carry.

If you are a caregiver reading this and feeling angry at the unwell parent, I understand that too. Anger is often grief in motion. But before you let anger become the story your child drinks every day, pause and remember: contempt will not stabilize a child. Dignity will. Truth will. Structure will. And steady love will.

In the end, honoring a parent who is unwell is not a sentimental idea. It is a stabilizing practice. It protects a child's identity. It protects family connection where connection can be safely preserved. And it helps children grow into adults who can hold complicated realities with compassion and strength. That is part of how a legacy of stability is built, one truthful, dignifying sentence at a time.

Legacy Takeaway

Honor is dignity, not denial. Children thrive when adults tell the truth with tenderness, protect safety with wise boundaries, and refuse to make any parent "junk" in the family story.

Next Step

Write a simple, age-appropriate script your child can hear repeatedly: (1) "You are safe," (2) "You did not cause this," (3) "You cannot fix it," and (4) "Your parent is valuable, and we have a plan." Practice saying it calmly when emotions rise.

Toolkit link:

Tool #7 — Child Dignity Script + Tool #19 — Role Drift Checklist (Kids Staying Kids).

Closing Prayer

God, give me wisdom to protect children with courage and tenderness. Help me tell the truth without contempt and set boundaries without breaking dignity. Teach our family to honor parents even when they are unwell, and to keep children free from adult burdens. Strengthen our home with steady love, wise structure, and grace that holds complicated stories. Amen.

Chapter 8
A Community That Holds: Why Support Networks Are Essential

One of the quiet lies mental illness tells a family is this: "You need to keep this private." Sometimes that lie comes from shame. Sometimes it comes from fear of judgment. Sometimes it comes from the family's desire to protect the person who is struggling. And sometimes it comes from exhaustion—because it feels easier to carry the load alone than to explain the story again and again.

But isolation never makes mental illness easier. It makes it heavier.

This is why the Community Anchor matters. A healthy support network is not optional for long-term stability. It is essential. Families need belonging. They need practical help. They need people who can show up without trying to fix. They need safe spaces where the story is not treated as scandal. And they need a community that understands the difference between spiritual care and clinical care—so support stays wise instead of harmful.

I want to say something that protects both faith communities and families: the Church cannot replace psychiatrists or therapists. And psychiatrists and therapists cannot replace a loving community. When each stays in its lane, healing becomes more sustainable. When one tries to become all lanes, people burn out, care gets sloppy, and families can feel abandoned or blamed.

In many faith communities, mental illness has historically been misunderstood. People were told they just needed more faith, more prayer, more discipline, more deliverance. And while prayer is powerful and faith is real, mental illness is also real. The brain is a physical organ. When it is unhealthy or injured, it affects stability, behavior, and connection. Families need communities that can hold both truths at the same time: we pray, and we pursue proper care.

A healthy community anchor does a few things exceptionally well.

First, it provides belonging without interrogation. People struggling with mental illness and the families who love them need to know they can show up and still be seen as valuable. They need to be greeted like humans, not like projects. They need to be included even when they are not "easy."

Second, it provides practical support. Meals, rides, childcare, a check-in text, a person who can sit with a child during a difficult week—these are not small things. These are stabilizers. Practical love lowers the pressure inside the home and protects caregiver capacity.

Third, it provides wise spiritual care. That means prayer that comforts instead of condemns. Scripture that strengthens instead of shames. Ministry that respects professional treatment instead of competing with it. It also means knowing when to refer. A healthy community can say, "We love you, and we will walk with you—and we also want you connected to clinical and medical support."

Fourth, it provides connection and purpose. Remember, these are non-negotiables. Community can offer meaningful roles that fit capacity: a small volunteer task, a creative outlet, a team that welcomes someone, a safe group where people can be honest. Purpose does not have to be public to be powerful. Many people stabilize when they feel they still belong and still contribute.

Now let me name the hard part. Not every community is healthy. Some communities gossip. Some minimize. Some spiritualize everything. Some panic at symptoms. Some reject families because they don't know what to do. If that has been your experience, I am sorry. And I want you to hear this: you are allowed to be discerning. You are allowed to choose a community that can hold your story with maturity.

Discerning community is also a boundary issue. You do not owe everyone full access to your story. You can share wisely. You can start small. You can choose one or two safe people before you share broadly. You can ask for specific help instead of telling every detail. Community support is not about exposure; it is about connection.

This is also where we protect the children again. Children benefit from safe community. They benefit from stable adults who can love them when parents are tired. They benefit from mentors and trusted friends who show them what steady love looks like. They benefit from a circle that says, "You are not alone."

And when a family is carrying long-term illness patterns, community is one of the ways you keep the home team from collapsing. This is where rotating support can extend beyond the family: one friend can check in weekly, another can help with transportation, another can provide respite, another can simply pray and stay present. The goal is not to create dependency. The goal is to create sustainability.

If you want a simple way to evaluate your community anchor, ask these questions: Do we feel safe here? Do we feel respected? Do people honor our dignity? Do they avoid shame language? Do they understand their lane? Do they help practically? Do they protect confidentiality? If the answer is yes more often than no, you may have found a community that can hold.

A community that holds is one of God's most practical gifts. It becomes a living reminder that you were never meant to do this alone. And when community is healthy, it doesn't just support the person who is unwell—it supports the whole family system. That is how stability becomes possible over the long haul.

Legacy Takeaway

Isolation makes illness heavier. A healthy support network provides belonging, practical help, and wise spiritual care—so stability becomes sustainable for the whole family.

Next Step

Identify one 'safe person' or 'safe circle' you can invite into your support plan. Ask for one specific, practical form of help (a check-in, a meal, childcare, a ride, or prayer support). Keep the ask clear and doable.

Toolkit link:

Tool #2 — Community Support Menu (How to Ask) + Tool #20 — Discerning Healthy Community Questions

Closing Prayer

God, help us step out of isolation and into wise support. Give us courage to ask for help, discernment to choose safe community, and humility to receive what we need. Teach our faith communities to hold mental illness with compassion and maturity. Surround our family with people who honor dignity, protect confidentiality, and strengthen stability through steady love. Amen.

Chapter 9
Managing Behavior Without Becoming the Diagnosis Manual

By this point in the book, you may be noticing something intentional: I'm not trying to turn you into a clinician. I'm not trying to make you memorize labels. And I'm not building a diagnosis manual with a Christian wrapper.

Why? Because most families don't need more labels. They need a way to manage what they are living with—day after day—without losing themselves, without losing each other, and without losing the child's sense of safety.

I'm not opposed to diagnosis. Diagnosis can be helpful. It can open doors to treatment, insurance coverage, and specific clinical tools. It can bring relief to a person who has felt confused for years. But diagnosis is not the same as daily management. And many families get stuck because they learn the label but don't learn the plan.

So this chapter is about a different approach. It is about managing behaviors and patterns in a way that is practical, dignifying, and sustainable—regardless of the diagnosis. It is about families learning how to respond to what is happening in front of them without becoming trapped in constant analysis.

Let me give you the framework I use with families. Most destabilizing behaviors fall into a few lived-out categories: escalation, shutdown, avoidance, impulsivity, and relational disruption. Different diagnoses can produce similar patterns. And similar patterns can be managed with similar stabilizing responses—while still respecting the individual's unique story.

Escalation is when the nervous system goes high: anger, agitation, rapid speech, yelling, blaming, threats, intense emotion, argument spirals. In escalation, the goal is not to win. The goal is to lower intensity, protect safety, and postpone problem-solving until regulation returns. That is why we practiced co-regulation and boundaries. Escalation is managed with calm tone, clear limits, reduced stimulation, and a plan that prevents "mutual destruction conversations."

Shutdown is the opposite: the nervous system goes low. People disappear emotionally. They go numb, silent, withdrawn, or frozen. Families often misread shutdown as stubbornness or passive aggression. But many times, shutdown is overwhelm. The brain is protecting itself by going offline. In shutdown, the goal is not to force engagement. The goal is to create safety and time, and then offer gentle reconnection without pressure. Shutdown is managed with low-demand connection, predictable rhythm, and compassionate invitations rather than interrogation.

Avoidance is when a person avoids responsibilities, treatment, conversations, accountability, or life tasks. Avoidance can be rooted in fear, shame, trauma, depression, anxiety, or simple immaturity. Families often try to solve avoidance with lectures. But lectures rarely build capacity. Avoidance is managed with clear expectations, supportive structure, and small steps that match capacity. It is also managed by the clinical anchor—because avoidance often needs skill-building and internal work, not just external pressure.

Impulsivity shows up as sudden decisions, risky behavior, overspending, substance use, sexual acting out, aggression, or drastic shifts in plans. Families often respond with panic and control. But control battles can inflame impulsivity. Impulsivity is managed with guardrails built in calm seasons: financial boundaries, safety agreements, supervision plans, accountability supports, and early warning sign tracking. This is where the crisis plan and the contact list protect the home.

Relational disruption is the pattern where the illness becomes relational warfare: triangulation, blame cycles, manipulation, testing love, loyalty conflicts, or repeated ruptures without repair. This is where connection and purpose become non-negotiable. The goal is not to tolerate harm. The goal is to build repair pathways, stop role drift, protect children from adult conflict, and keep dignity intact while requiring safe behavior.

Now here is the biggest shift families need: stop asking, "What is wrong with you?" and start asking, "What is happening in the system right now?" That question moves you from personal attack to collaborative care. It helps you remember the Anchors. It helps you choose the right lane. It keeps you from becoming the family detective.

It also helps you avoid a common trap: over-accommodating. Many families, trying to be compassionate, remove every discomfort from the person who is struggling. They lower expectations to zero. They rearrange the entire household around symptoms. They allow chaos because they're afraid of making things worse. That is not compassion. That is collapse.

Compassion with structure says: "We will make room for what is real, and we will also build what is needed." We will match expectations to capacity without removing responsibility completely. We will support treatment without doing treatment for you. We will protect children without teaching contempt.

We will hold boundaries without breaking connection.

So what does this look like day to day? It looks like a family noticing patterns early, using agreed-upon scripts, and moving toward support quickly. It looks like asking, "Which category are we in right now—escalation, shutdown, avoidance, impulsivity, or relational disruption?" Then you respond with the matching stabilizing move. You don't have to diagnose to respond wisely.

This is especially important for caregivers who are exhausted. When you are tired, you don't have energy for complicated frameworks. You need a simple map. This chapter is your map. It keeps you from being pulled into the endless question of labels and it moves you toward the practical question of response.

In the next chapters, we will begin to build more specific tools—communication scripts, repair practices, and family agreements. But I want you to carry this foundation: behavior can be understood without contempt. Patterns can be managed without becoming a label manual. And stability can grow when families learn to respond with calm, structure, and shared support.

Legacy Takeaway

You don't have to become a diagnosis expert to respond wisely. When families manage lived-out behavior patterns with calm structure and shared support, stability grows without shame.

Next Step

Use the 'pattern categories' for one week. When things get tense, ask: Are we in escalation, shutdown, avoidance, impulsivity, or relational disruption? Choose one matching stabilizing move and write down what helped.

Toolkit link:

Tool #3 — Behavior Pattern Map (5 Categories) + Tool #21 — Matching Response Scripts

Closing Prayer

God, give me wisdom to respond to what we are living with—without fear, without contempt, and without shame. Help me see patterns clearly and choose steady, practical steps that protect safety, dignity, connection, and purpose. Teach our family to build structure that holds and support that is shared, so love can endure. Amen.

Chapter 10
Listening That Lowers the Temperature: Communication as a Stabilizing Skill

If you've lived with mental illness in a family system, you already know this: communication is rarely just about information. It's about safety. It's about power. It's about fear. It's about shame. And in a home under strain, conversations can become the place where pain spills out sideways.

Most families don't need to become perfect communicators. They need a few reliable skills that consistently lower the temperature. They need a way to talk without escalating. They need a way to hear each other without interrupting. And they need a way to repair after hard moments so the home doesn't become a museum of unresolved conflict.

I'm going to say something that brings hope: listening is a skill. It is not a personality trait. Some people may have a natural gift for empathy, but every single person can learn to listen better. And in families carrying mental illness, active listening is one of the most stabilizing practices you can build.

Here is why. When a nervous system feels unheard, it gets louder. When someone feels misunderstood, they often intensify—through anger, withdrawal, blame, or accusation. But when a person feels genuinely heard, the nervous system begins to downshift. Listening doesn't solve everything, but it reduces the intensity that makes everything harder.

Active listening has three simple movements: receive, reflect, and respond.

Receive means you stop preparing your rebuttal while the other person is speaking. This is harder than it sounds, especially for responsible caregivers who are used to managing problems. But receiving is the act of honoring. It says, "Your experience matters enough for me to fully hear it."

Reflect means you mirror back what you heard in your own words. Not as a sarcastic echo, but as a genuine check-in: "What I'm hearing is…" or "It sounds like you're feeling…" Reflection slows the conversation down and reduces misunderstanding. It also gives the speaker a chance to clarify without escalating.

Respond means you choose a next step that fits the moment. Sometimes the response is empathy: "That makes sense." Sometimes the response is curiosity: "Help me understand what part felt most threatening." Sometimes the response is a boundary: "I'm willing to talk, but not while we're yelling." And sometimes the response is a pause: "I need ten minutes to settle so I can stay kind."

Notice what active listening is not. It is not agreeing with everything someone says. You can reflect someone's feelings and still disagree with their conclusions. You can validate emotion without validating harmful behavior. You can honor a person while still holding a boundary.

This matters because in families affected by mental illness, conversations often get tangled in blame. People say things they don't mean. They interpret tone as threat. They assume motives. They react to old wounds. If you can build one or two listening habits that slow things down, you reduce the amount of relational damage that has to be repaired later.

Now let's talk about timing, because timing is a communication tool.

Many families try to resolve serious issues in the exact moment emotions are hottest. That is like trying to do surgery during an earthquake. Your goal in a heated moment is not full resolution. Your goal is safety and downshifting. You can say, "This matters. We will talk. But we will talk when we are calm." That sentence alone has saved many homes from a spiral.

A helpful phrase I teach families is: "We can be connected without being resolved." Connection means we stay respectful, we don't threaten the relationship, and we don't turn disagreement into war. Resolution can wait. Most decisions can wait until the nervous system is regulated.

And yes, this is where the home team may need to rotate leadership again. If one person is more easily triggered, another person may take the lead in de-escalation. If one person is more skillful at staying calm, they may become the "temperature setter" in the room. This is not about superiority. It's about stewardship of capacity and skill.

Let's talk about kids for a moment. Children learn communication by watching adults. If they grow up in a home where conflict is handled with contempt, they learn contempt. If they grow up in a home where people repair after rupture, they learn repair. This is one of the most powerful legacy gifts you can give: teaching a child that hard conversations can be handled with dignity.

So what does repair look like? Repair is a short, honest return to connection after rupture. It can sound like: "I was sharp. I'm sorry." "I raised my voice. That wasn't okay." "I got defensive. I'm willing to try again." "I care about you, and I want us to be okay." Repair does not require a long speech. It requires humility and consistency.

Families sometimes resist repair because they think it excuses the behavior. It doesn't. Repair strengthens the relationship so boundaries and accountability can actually be heard. In a disconnected home, boundaries feel like attacks. In a connected home, boundaries feel like guardrails.

If you are thinking, "This sounds great, but my person won't listen," remember: you can only control your lane. You can still practice active listening with other adults in the system. You can still model calm. You can still refuse to escalate. And you can still strengthen the Anchors of Support so communication skills are taught and reinforced clinically as well.

Communication is one of the top reasons relationships fracture under strain. That's not because families are bad. It's because stress changes the nervous system. But skills can be learned. And when skills are learned, the home gets steadier. That is the goal of this chapter: a few reliable habits that make hard conversations safer—so love can last.

Legacy Takeaway

Listening is a stabilizing skill. When families learn to receive, reflect, and respond—with wise timing and repair—conflict stops ruling the home.

Next Step

Practice one active listening habit this week: reflect before you respond. Use the phrase, "What I'm hearing is…" once per day in a conversation that matters. If emotions rise, add one timing boundary: "This matters. Let's talk when we're calm."

Toolkit link:

Tool #10 — Active Listening Script + Tool #22 — Repair Phrases (Short + True)

Closing Prayer

God, teach me to listen with patience and respond with wisdom. Help our home slow down when emotions rise, speak truth with dignity, and repair quickly when we miss each other. Give us courage to set boundaries that protect kindness, and grace to stay connected even when we are not yet resolved. Make our conversations a place of safety, not war, and let steady communication strengthen our legacy of stability. Amen.

Chapter 11
Caregiver Capacity: Rotating the Lead and Renegotiating the Plan

If you have been the responsible one in a family system touched by mental illness, you know the quiet exhaustion I'm talking about. You're the one who notices the warning signs first. You're the one who remembers the appointments. You're the one who keeps the bills paid, the kids steady, the groceries stocked, and the crisis contained. You're the one who keeps life moving while everyone else reacts.

And because you can do it, people assume you should do it.

But capacity is not endless. Capacity is a stewardship issue. And if we ignore capacity, we end up with two crises instead of one: the person who is struggling becomes unstable, and the caregiver collapses under the weight of being the whole system.

This is why I keep returning to the same principle: long-term stability requires a structure that can be renegotiated as life changes. What worked in one season may fail in the next. What you used to be able to carry may become impossible after grief, aging, medical issues, burnout, or simply the accumulation of years of strain. That does not mean you are weak. It means you are human.

One of the most practical ways families protect capacity is by rotating the lead caregiver. Rotating the lead doesn't mean rotating love. It means rotating responsibility so the system stays strong.

Here is what rotating the lead can look like in real life. In one season, one adult is the primary appointment coordinator. In another season, someone else becomes the point person with the clinician or prescriber. One person may handle daily routines because they are naturally structured. Another may handle crisis de-escalation because they stay calm under pressure. Another may take the role of 'community connector'—the one who asks for practical support when the family is tired. The roles don't have to be equal. They just have to be shared wisely.

Some families hear that and think, "That's great, but I don't have anyone else." I understand. Not every family has multiple adults available. Some caregivers are single parents. Some are the only stable adult in the system. Some are caring for a spouse who is unwell while also caring for children. In those situations, rotating the lead may mean rotating with community support—trusted friends, extended family, faith community, respite services, or professional supports. The principle is the same: you cannot be the entire system alone.

Capacity also requires honest assessment. Many caregivers stay in denial about depletion because they think love means constant availability. But constant availability is not love; it is unsustainable. And unsustainable love becomes resentment, numbness, or burnout. This is where we replace guilt with wisdom.

Here are a few signs your capacity needs renegotiation: you feel dread most mornings; you are consistently irritable or emotionally flat; you are losing sleep; you are forgetting things; you are constantly anxious; you have little compassion left; you fantasize about disappearing; you feel like you're living in emergency mode even when the day is calm. Those are not moral failures. Those are signals.

When you notice those signals, the question becomes: what needs to shift? Sometimes the shift is practical. You reduce commitments. You simplify schedules. You ask for help. You create more predictable rhythms. You tighten boundaries. You protect sleep. You schedule regular respite. Sometimes the shift is clinical. You get your own counselor because caregiving creates trauma exposure, grief, and chronic stress. Sometimes the shift is spiritual. You stop pretending you're okay and begin receiving care, prayer, and companionship.

Renegotiation also protects the person who is struggling. When caregivers are depleted, they often become either controlling or permissive. They clamp down because they're scared, or they collapse boundaries because they're tired. Neither response builds stability. When caregivers regain capacity, they can hold the middle: compassion with structure. They can hold boundaries with bridges. They can maintain connection and purpose without becoming the caretaker of every emotion.

This is also a place where families need a 'permission statement.' A permission statement is a sentence you give yourself when guilt rises. Here are a few examples: "I am allowed to rest." "I am allowed to need help." "I am allowed to protect my health." "I am allowed to say no without abandoning love." "I am allowed to renegotiate what I can carry." Guilt will argue with those statements, but truth must lead.

Let's bring children back into the picture, because caregiver capacity affects kids directly. When the responsible adult is depleted, children often become hyper-aware and anxious. They sense the fragility in the system. They may try to be perfect to reduce stress. Or they may act out because their nervous system is overloaded. Protecting your capacity is one

of the most child-centered things you can do—
because your steadiness becomes their stability.

And finally, capacity requires humility. Some families
resist renegotiation because they want to be the hero.
They want to prove they can handle it. But this book
is built on a different thesis: you cannot manage
mental illness as a dominant. It takes shared support.
It takes a community of care. And the strongest
families are not the ones who carry the most alone.
The strongest families are the ones who build a
structure that holds over time.

So if you're the responsible one, let me speak to you
gently: your role matters. Your steadiness matters.
But you were never meant to be the whole plan. This
chapter is your invitation to build something
sustainable—a caregiving structure that can breathe,
flex, and endure. That is how you protect the legacy.
Not by carrying more. By carrying wiser.

Legacy Takeaway

Capacity is stewardship. Rotating the lead and
renegotiating roles protects the caregiver, stabilizes
the home, and prevents the system from collapsing
under chronic strain.

Next Step

Complete a quick capacity check: list (1) what you are carrying that is truly yours, (2) what can be shared with another anchor or person, and (3) one commitment you can reduce this month. Then choose one role to rotate or one support to add.

Toolkit link:

Tool #18 — Caregiver Capacity Check + Tool #23 — Role Rotation Map

Closing Prayer

God, give me wisdom to steward my capacity with humility and courage. Help me release what I was never meant to carry alone, and show me how to build shared support that is sustainable. Strengthen me to love with structure, set boundaries with grace, and protect the children and vulnerable in our care. Renew my strength, restore my joy, and help our family endure with steady love. Amen.

Chapter 12
The Living Plan: Family Agreements That Can Be Renegotiated

By now, you've heard me say it several times because it's central to this entire framework: long-term stability requires a structure that can be renegotiated as life changes.

That sentence is not just a nice idea. It is a survival tool for families. Because one of the reasons homes collapse under the weight of mental illness is that families build a plan for one season and then try to live in that same plan forever. They don't adjust when capacity changes. They don't update roles as kids grow. They don't revise routines when symptoms shift. They don't renegotiate expectations when aging parents, new jobs, financial stress, or health issues enter the story.

So this chapter is where we get very practical: you need a living plan. Not a complicated binder. Not a stack of papers no one reads. A living plan is a simple, shared agreement that everyone can point to when emotions get loud. It brings clarity to the home. It reduces power struggles. And it prevents the responsible person from being the only one carrying the mental load.

A living plan answers four questions.

First: what are we building? This is where you name your main thing. In this book, our main thing is a legacy of stability—connection and purpose protected, safety and dignity held, and support shared. When families name what they are building, they stop fighting over small issues as if they are the whole story.

Second: who does what? This is where you bring back the Anchors and the lanes. Who is the Clinical Anchor? Who is the Medical Anchor? Who is the Community Anchor? Who is on the Home Team, and what roles are shared? The plan does not have to be equal. It has to be clear.

Third: what are the non-negotiables in this home? Non-negotiables are the guardrails that protect what is sacred. In many families, non-negotiables include: no yelling at children, no threats, no intimidation, no violence, no substance use in the home, no driving impaired, no using kids as messengers, no adult conflict in front of kids, and no breaking boundaries through manipulation. Your non-negotiables must fit your real situation. The goal is not perfection. The goal is safety and dignity.

Fourth: how do we respond when things get hard? This is where your crisis plan, your listening skills, your boundary scripts, and your role-rotation plans become real. It is where you decide ahead of time what you will do when escalation, shutdown, avoidance, impulsivity, or relational disruption show up. The living plan doesn't just describe your values. It gives you a pathway back to stability.

Now, here is where many families get stuck: they think a family agreement requires everyone to be emotionally mature and cooperative. It doesn't. A living plan can start with the people who are willing. In fact, it often has to. The responsible adult may be the one who begins. A grandparent may begin. A co-parent may begin. A support team may begin. The plan can still protect children and stabilize the home even if the struggling person is not fully participating yet.

That said, when possible, it is powerful to invite the person who is struggling into the plan in a regulated season. Not as a courtroom meeting. As a partnership conversation. The tone matters. It sounds like: "I love you. I want us to have more peace. Can we build a plan for hard days so we don't destroy each other when stress rises?"

When families do this, something beautiful often happens: the plan stops feeling like control and starts feeling like relief. Many people living with mental illness are tired too. They are tired of being ashamed. Tired of being misunderstood. Tired of apologizing. Tired of losing relationships. A living plan can become a form of hope: "We are not giving up on you, and we are not giving up on us."

Let me also say this clearly: the living plan must include the caregiver's capacity. If your plan assumes unlimited energy from one person, it will fail. That is why rotating the lead is not optional. It is part of the agreement. The plan should include: how we will share the load, when we will ask for help, and what respite looks like. This protects the caregiver and it protects the whole system.

And yes—this is where community matters again. A living plan is stronger when the family has at least one or two outside supports who know the plan at a basic level. Not the private details, but the essentials. Who to call. What the boundaries are. What the child safety plan is. Where the escalation line sits. Support cannot help you if they don't know what you need.

If you are a person of faith, you can also include spiritual practices in your plan as stabilizers—not as magic fixes, but as rhythm. Prayer as a daily anchor. Worship as a nervous-system reset. Scripture as a reminder of dignity and hope. Community as belonging. These are not replacements for clinical care. They are supports that strengthen the whole person.

Finally, a living plan must be revisited. Renegotiation is not a failure. Renegotiation is wisdom. Set a simple rhythm: review the plan every month for three months, then quarterly, and anytime there is a major shift (hospitalization, medication changes, relapse, job changes, family transitions, or capacity shifts). Keep asking: what is working, what is not working, and what needs to be updated?

This is how families build stability over time—not through one perfect plan, but through faithful adjustments. A living plan keeps the home from drifting. It keeps children safer. It keeps caregivers from collapsing. It keeps dignity intact. And it keeps connection and purpose within reach, even when the story is complicated.

Legacy Takeaway

A living plan turns values into stability. Clear roles, non-negotiables, and a shared response pathway protect the home—and the plan can be renegotiated as life changes.

Next Step

Draft a one-page Family Living Plan with four headings: (1) What we're building, (2) Who does what (Anchors + Home Team roles), (3) Our non-negotiables, and (4) Our response pathway when things get hard. Review it with one trusted adult this week.

Toolkit link:

Tool #24 — Family Living Plan (One Page) + Tool #25 — Non-Negotiables Builder

Closing Prayer

God, give our family wisdom to build a plan that holds. Help us live with clear roles, strong boundaries, and steady love. Teach us to protect what is sacred—especially children—while honoring dignity and keeping connection open. Give us courage to ask for help, humility to share the load, and grace to renegotiate our plan as life changes. Let our home become a place of stability and hope. Amen.

Chapter 13
Situational Storm or Long-Term Illness: Knowing What You're Dealing With

One of the most confusing things for families is trying to figure out what kind of struggle they're facing. Is this a situational storm—grief, trauma, postpartum changes, job loss, a breakup, medical illness, a season of overwhelm? Or is this a long-term, diagnosable mental illness that will require ongoing clinical and medical care?

That question matters because families often respond in extremes. If they assume everything is just "a tough season," they may delay treatment, minimize warning signs, or spiritualize what needs medical attention. If they assume everything is a lifelong diagnosis, they may panic, catastrophize, and lose hope before they even have accurate information. Neither extreme brings stability.

So let's build a wiser middle: we respond to what we see, we get proper evaluation, and we hold our conclusions with humility until we have clarity.

Here is the first principle: symptoms are real whether they are situational or long-term. A panic attack is real. A depressive episode is real. A trauma response is real. Sleep collapse is real. Emotional regression is real. Suicidal thinking is real. The question is not "Is it real?" The question is "What is driving it, what is the pattern over time, and what level of support is needed?"

Situational mental health crises often have a clear trigger: a death, a betrayal, a move, a major medical diagnosis, a traumatic event, childbirth, financial collapse, loss of identity, or a season of relentless stress. The nervous system can get overloaded, and symptoms can be intense. People may look "not like themselves." Families may feel shocked. But when the trigger is addressed and proper support is added, the person often stabilizes over time.

Long-term mental illness can also be triggered or intensified by stress, but it usually shows a broader pattern: symptoms that recur across seasons, symptoms that persist beyond the original trigger, symptoms that affect functioning in multiple areas (work, relationships, sleep, self-care), and symptoms that require ongoing treatment management. Long-term illness may also have a family history component, early life trauma, brain-based vulnerabilities, or chronic dysregulation that does not simply resolve when circumstances improve.

Now, let me say this carefully: families are not responsible to diagnose. Clinicians diagnose. Prescribers diagnose. Your job is to observe patterns, protect safety, and pursue proper evaluation.

This is why the Medical Anchor matters so much. Sometimes what looks like mental illness is a medical issue: thyroid imbalance, hormone shifts, sleep disorders, neurological issues, medication side effects, substance interactions, nutritional deficiencies, chronic pain, infections, or other conditions that affect mood and cognition. Families can waste years trying to "counsel" something that requires medical investigation. Medical evaluation is not lack of faith. It is wisdom.

And the Clinical Anchor matters because whether the issue is situational or long-term, people need skills. They need emotional regulation tools. They need trauma processing when trauma is present. They need relational skills and boundaries. They need support to rebuild rhythms. A therapist or counselor can help differentiate what is stress-driven and what is deeper, and they can help the family build a plan either way.

So how do you tell the difference in real life? You don't tell the difference by guessing. You tell the difference by tracking.

Tracking doesn't have to be complicated. It can be a simple weekly check-in where you note: sleep, appetite, energy, mood swings, irritability, isolation, impulsivity, substance use, functioning at work or school, and relational stability. Over time, patterns become clearer. Tracking also helps clinicians and prescribers make better decisions. It moves the conversation from vague statements—"They're acting crazy again"—to specific observations—"Sleep dropped to three hours for five nights, speech became rapid, spending increased, and conflict escalated."

Tracking also helps families avoid moralizing. When families moralize symptoms, they tend to shame the person. They assume laziness. They assume selfishness. They assume bad character. But when families track patterns, they start to see the nervous system at work. They start to see what intensifies symptoms and what stabilizes them. That's where compassion and structure become possible.

Now, here is the other truth we must hold: even situational storms can require intensive support. A person can experience a temporary crisis that still needs medication, hospitalization, or structured care for a season. And long-term illness can have seasons of calm. So do not equate "intensity" with "lifelong." And do not equate "calm" with "cured." That's why the living plan must be renegotiated as life changes.

I also want to name something families rarely talk about: the grief of not knowing. The in-between season can feel exhausting. You are waiting for clarity. You are watching for patterns. You are trying to protect the children. You are trying to keep work going. You are trying to keep hope alive. In that season, your job is not to predict the future. Your job is to build the Anchors and protect stability today.

So let this be your anchor sentence for this chapter: we do not need a perfect label to take wise action. We need observation, evaluation, and a plan.

That approach keeps you from becoming a diagnosis manual. It keeps you from minimizing reality. It keeps you from catastrophizing. And it helps you build a home that responds to what is true with courage, wisdom, and steady love.

Legacy Takeaway

You don't need a perfect label to take wise action. Track patterns, pursue proper evaluation, and build support that fits what you're living—whether the storm is situational or long-term.

Next Step

Start a simple weekly tracking note for 6 weeks: sleep, mood, energy, functioning, conflict level, and any major triggers. Bring your notes to your clinician/prescriber to support clearer evaluation and planning.

Toolkit link:

Tool #6 — Weekly Pattern Tracker (6 Weeks) + Tool #11 — Questions to Ask a Clinician/Prescriber

Closing Prayer

God, give us wisdom to see clearly and respond wisely. Help us avoid minimizing what is real and avoid fear that outruns the facts. Guide us toward proper evaluation, steady support, and a plan that protects safety, dignity, connection, and purpose. Give us patience in the in-between season and courage to take the next right step. Amen.

Chapter 14
The Age of Our Wounds: Understanding Emotional Regression

Sometimes the hardest moments in a family are not the loud ones. They're the confusing ones—the moments when a grown adult suddenly seems like a frightened child, a defiant teenager, or someone who cannot access the maturity you know they carry in other situations. [2][3][4]

You try logic. You try reason. You try to explain. And nothing lands.

If you've ever stood in that moment and thought, "Why are they acting like this?" I want to give you a framework that can change how you respond: they may not be responding as the age they are now—they may be responding as the age of their wound.

This is what we call emotional regression. It isn't someone "being childish" for attention. It's often a nervous system dropping into survival mode. Under stress, the brain can reach for an older pattern that was formed when the person first learned that the world was unsafe, unpredictable, or shaming. In that moment, they are not performing. They are reliving.

Let's make it practical. A person who was abandoned at five may feel panic when someone leaves the room. A person who was shamed for expressing emotion may become angry or numb when they feel vulnerable. A person who grew up in criticism may spiral when they receive even gentle feedback. To the family, it looks disproportionate. To the nervous system, it feels like the original danger is happening again.

This is why regression can become so disorienting for loved ones. You're talking to the adult in your mind, but their body is responding from a younger place.

There is also a neurological reason this happens. Under threat, the brain's alarm system takes over. The rational, adult reasoning center can go offline temporarily, especially when someone is already depleted by poor sleep, chronic stress, trauma history, or a mental health condition. This is why you can't "argue" someone out of regression. Their logic center is not running the show in that moment.

So what do families do? The goal is not correction first. The goal is safety first.

Safety does not mean permissiveness. Safety means calm tone, grounded presence, and simple structure. It means you stop trying to win the conversation and start trying to lower the temperature. It means you protect dignity by not correcting someone publicly, not shaming them, and not escalating with your own fear.

This is where co-regulation becomes a gift. Your calm nervous system can help their nervous system downshift. That does not mean you absorb their chaos. It means you stay anchored. You breathe slower. You speak gentler. You keep your words short. You offer simple choices. You say things like, "You're safe. I'm here. We can take a minute."

One of the most helpful shifts is learning to validate feelings without validating harmful behavior. Validation sounds like: "I can tell this feels really big for you." "I hear that you feel threatened." "I can see you're overwhelmed." Validation does not sound like: "You're right to scream." "It's okay to threaten." "You can talk to me however you want." Validation is emotional dignity. Boundaries are behavioral dignity. Healthy homes hold both.

Regression also requires timing. The moment is not the time to do deep processing. The moment is for downshifting and safety. After the nervous system settles, then you can gently ask, "What felt triggering?" Or, "What did you need in that moment?" And if the person has the capacity, you can also ask, "How old did you feel right then?" That one question can bring remarkable insight.

This is also where families protect children. Children can be confused and frightened when they see adult regression. They may assume they caused it. They may feel responsible to fix it. They may become hypervigilant. So we keep children out of the storm. We give them a simple script: "Mom/Dad is overwhelmed right now. You are safe. The adults are handling it." We do not recruit children to soothe an adult.

If you are the caregiver, I want to honor something: regression can be exhausting to witness. It can trigger your own wounds. It can tempt you toward anger, sarcasm, or control. This is why caregiver capacity matters. You cannot co-regulate well if you are depleted. Sometimes the wisest move is to step back, tag in another support person, and come back when you can be steady.

And sometimes, yes, regression needs clinical support. If emotional regression is frequent, intense, or connected to trauma, a skilled counselor can help the person build insight, develop regulation tools, and heal the underlying wound. Families can support, but they cannot replace trauma work.

I also want to name the faith layer here. Scripture gives us a picture of gentleness with the wounded. God does not shame bruised places. He protects them. He restores. He calls us to compassion that does not break dignity. When someone regresses, your gentleness can become a sacred environment—one where healing begins not with correction, but with safety.

So here is the anchor takeaway: when you recognize regression, you stop treating it like a character flaw and start treating it like a nervous system signal. You respond with calm, structure, and dignity. You lower the temperature first. Then you build insight later. That one shift can change the climate of a home—and it can keep relationship from breaking under the strain of misunderstood pain.

Legacy Takeaway

Emotional regression is often the nervous system responding from the age of an old wound. Safety first—then insight. Calm presence, clear boundaries, and dignifying language protect connection and stability.

Next Step

Choose one "downshift script" you will use in heated moments: "You're safe. I'm here. Let's take a minute." Pair it with one boundary: "I'm willing to talk when we're calm." After the moment passes, ask one gentle question: "What felt triggering?"

Toolkit link:

Tool #9 — Co-Regulation Scripts + Tool #26 — Emotional Regression Quick Guide (Do's/Don'ts)

Closing Prayer

God, give me gentleness when wounds show up loud. Help me respond with calm, dignity, and wise boundaries that protect what is sacred. Teach me to lower the temperature before I try to solve the problem, and help our family grow in understanding without shame. Bring healing to the places in us that still feel young and afraid, and let Your steady love shape stability in our home. Amen.

Chapter 15
Boundaries With Bridges:
Protecting Safety Without Breaking Connection

One of the most misunderstood words in families living with mental illness is boundaries. [5]

Some people hear boundaries and think control. Others hear boundaries and think rejection. Some families avoid boundaries because they feel unkind. Other families use boundaries like weapons—sharp, final, and punishing. Neither extreme builds stability.

In this book, we are aiming for something better: boundaries that protect what is sacred without breaking relationship connection, value, or purpose.

That sentence matters because many families have lived the painful cycle. Symptoms escalate. Everyone gets hurt. Someone draws a hard line in anger. Connection ruptures. Shame increases. And then the system becomes even more fragile because isolation grows. The child feels the tension. The caregiver feels guilt. The person who is struggling feels abandoned. Then the next crisis hits and the same cycle repeats.

Healthy boundaries interrupt that cycle.

A boundary is simply a clear limit that protects safety, dignity, and capacity. It answers the question: "What is okay in this home, and what is not?" It also answers: "What will I do if the line is crossed?" A boundary is not a demand that someone change. A boundary is what you will do to protect what is sacred if someone does not change.

That is why boundaries are not mean. They are stewardship.

But—this is important—boundaries work best when they are paired with bridges. A bridge is the relational pathway that keeps dignity and connection available when connection can be safely preserved. Boundaries without bridges often communicate, "You are a problem." Boundaries with bridges communicate, "You are valuable—and we are also protecting safety."

Let's make this practical.

A boundary might sound like: "I am willing to talk, but not while we are yelling." The bridge is: "I want to understand you, and I'll come back to this conversation when we're calm."

A boundary might be: "We will not allow substance use in the home." The bridge is: "We will help you pursue treatment, and you can be with us when you are sober and safe."

A boundary might be: "Children will not be exposed to adult conflict." The bridge is: "We will protect their hearts—and we will also keep dignity for both adults in the story."

A boundary might be: "We will not tolerate threats or intimidation." The bridge is: "We will call for support when safety is at risk, and we will return to the relationship when things are stable."

Now, let's talk about the 'yucky gut'—that internal signal many caregivers describe. When your stomach tightens, when you feel irritated and discombobulated, when you feel resentful or trapped, that is often a boundary check. It may mean you are giving someone more access, more space in your head, more of your time or emotional energy than you can handle. Or it may mean your home is absorbing stress that belongs in another anchor's lane.

Instead of ignoring that signal, use it as information. Ask: What boundary is being crossed? What do I need to clarify? What role drift is happening here? What support do we need to add so I'm not trying to do this alone?

Families also need to understand that boundaries protect capacity. If the caregiver's capacity collapses, the whole system becomes unstable. So sometimes the boundary is not about behavior; it is about bandwidth. It can sound like: "I can't do three appointments this week. We need to rotate the lead." Or: "I can't keep absorbing late-night crisis conversations. We need a plan for after-hours support."

This is where many families struggle: they set boundaries, but they do not follow through. They say, "If you do that again, we're done," but then the line is crossed and nothing changes. That creates more instability because the home loses credibility. People learn that boundaries are just emotional speeches.

So let me give you a simple rule: set fewer boundaries, but keep them. A boundary that you will actually follow through on is better than ten boundaries you cannot maintain.

It also helps to keep your boundaries calm and predictable. When boundaries are delivered in rage, they feel like punishment. When boundaries are delivered with steadiness, they feel like guardrails. And remember: the goal is not to win a boundary battle. The goal is to create a stable environment where connection and purpose can remain possible.

Now, a word for families who love someone who resists boundaries: your boundaries may be one of the most loving gifts you ever give. Some people only pursue treatment when the home stops accommodating chaos. Some people only face reality when their behaviors have consistent consequences. That is not cruelty. That is clarity.

But boundaries should never be used to humiliate or shame. Even when consequences are necessary, dignity matters. You can be firm without being cruel. You can be clear without being contemptuous. You can be honest without making someone "junk."

And if you are raising children in this environment, boundaries become one of the strongest ways you teach love. Children learn that love does not mean tolerating harm. They learn that love includes protection. They learn that adults can set limits without losing their humanity. That is a legacy thought a child can carry into adulthood.

So if boundaries have felt confusing, here is the simple framework: a boundary protects what is sacred; a bridge protects dignity and connection. You need both. And when you practice both with steadiness, the home becomes safer—not only physically, but emotionally. That is what stability feels like: clear lines, kind tone, and love that lasts.

Legacy Takeaway

Boundaries protect what is sacred. Bridges protect dignity and connection. Together, they create a home where safety and relationship can coexist.

Next Step

Choose one boundary your home needs most right now. Write it in one calm sentence, then add the bridge sentence that keeps dignity and connection available. Practice saying both without anger.

Toolkit link:

Tool #12 — Boundaries With Bridges Script + Tool #13 — The Yucky Gut Boundary Check

Closing Prayer

God, give me courage to set wise boundaries and humility to keep my tone kind. Teach me to protect what is sacred without breaking dignity or connection. Help our family build clear guardrails with steady follow-through, and show us how to keep bridges of love open whenever it is safe. Give us wisdom, peace, and strength as we build a legacy of stability. Amen.

Chapter 16
Compassionate Language: Reducing Shame and Strengthening Healing

Words shape nervous systems. In families carrying mental illness, language can either steady the room or light a match. Most caregivers don't mean to harm with words—they are tired, scared, and trying to survive. But when stress is high, we often default to phrases that sound like truth and feel like correction, yet land as shame.

Shame is not the same as accountability. Shame says, 'You are bad.' Accountability says, 'This behavior is not okay, and we need a plan.' Shame collapses motivation and increases hiding. Accountability, delivered with dignity, can actually invite change—because it keeps the person's value intact.

If you want one simple goal for language in a strained home, let it be this: speak in a way that protects dignity while still telling the truth. Dignity doesn't mean softness without limits. It means we refuse to turn a person into a problem, even while we name what is unsafe or unsustainable.

Here are common 'shame phrases' families use—often without realizing it—and healthier alternatives that preserve dignity and still hold reality:

- 'What is wrong with you?' → 'What's happening for you right now?'
- 'You're being crazy.' → 'This feels intense. Let's slow down.'
- 'Just calm down.' → 'I can see you're flooded. Let's take a minute.'
- 'You always do this.' → 'I'm noticing a pattern, and we need a plan.'
- 'You're ruining everything.' → 'This is affecting the whole house. We have to protect safety.'
- 'If you loved us, you'd stop.' → 'I believe you love us, and we still need treatment and boundaries.'

Compassionate language is not word-policing. It is pattern-breaking. When you shift language, you shift the emotional climate, which makes it easier for every anchor to function: clinicians can build skills, medical providers can adjust care with better information, community can support without stigma, and the home team can hold boundaries without contempt.

Compassionate language also protects the children. Kids don't just hear what you say about the unwell parent—they hear what you say about human struggle. If a child learns that illness equals contempt, they may hide their own struggles later. If a child learns that truth and dignity can coexist, they gain a life-long framework for faith, relationships, and resilience.

One more important distinction: compassion does not mean you explain everything away as illness. Families can accidentally erase responsibility by saying, 'It's not them, it's the diagnosis.' But people are still agents. A healthier frame is: 'The illness is real, and choices still matter.' That sentence allows you to require treatment follow-through, safe behavior, and repair—without turning the person into a villain.

Practically, compassionate language works best when it is paired with two other things you've already built: timing and boundaries. If the nervous system is flooded, keep words short. If safety is at risk, move to your plan. If the person is regulated, you can have fuller conversations. The goal is not perfect sentences. The goal is a home where truth is spoken without cruelty and limits are held without contempt.

Legacy Takeaway

Language either increases shame or strengthens stability. When families use dignifying, truthful words, accountability becomes possible without collapsing connection.

Next Step

Choose three shame phrases you tend to use under stress. Write your replacement phrases and practice them when you're calm, so they are available when you're tired.

Toolkit link:

Tool #27 — Compassionate Language Swap List (Shame → Dignity)

Closing Prayer

God, set a guard over my mouth and give me words that heal instead of harm. Teach me to tell the truth with dignity, to hold boundaries without contempt, and to speak in a way that protects the vulnerable—especially children. When I am tired and afraid, slow me down. Let my language build safety, strengthen connection, and support healing in our home. Amen.

Chapter 17
Repair After Rupture: Rebuilding Trust Without Denial

Mental illness can create repeated ruptures—blowups, withdrawals, broken promises, missed responsibilities, harsh words, and seasons where the home feels like it is walking on glass. Families often respond to rupture in two unhealthy ways: they pretend it didn't happen to keep the peace, or they rehearse it endlessly until the relationship becomes a courtroom.

Repair is the wiser middle. Repair is not denial, and repair is not punishment. Repair is a structured return to connection after something has gone wrong. It names reality, restores dignity, and rebuilds trust one small step at a time.

Why is repair so important? Because a home without repair becomes a home with accumulation. Hurt piles up. People become guarded. Children become anxious. Caregivers become hardened. And the person who is struggling often begins to believe, 'I always ruin things,' which fuels more shame and more instability.

Repair is a skill, and it can be taught. The simplest repair has four parts:

1) Name what happened (briefly). 'I raised my voice.' 'I threatened.' 'I disappeared for two days.'
2) Name the impact. 'That scared you.' 'That disrupted the kids.' 'That damaged trust.'
3) Take responsibility for your part. 'That wasn't okay.' 'I own that.'
4) Name the next step. 'Here's what I'll do next time.' 'Here's the boundary we need.' 'Here's the support I'm adding.'

Notice what is missing: a long speech, a defense, or a demand that the other person 'move on.' Repair is not about managing someone's feelings. It is about restoring safety and credibility.

Families sometimes ask, 'But what if the person keeps repeating the same behavior?' Then repair must include the living plan. Repair without change becomes manipulation—apologies that reset consequences without building stability. But change doesn't have to be dramatic to be real. Change can be: making the therapy appointment, taking medication as prescribed, using the crisis plan earlier, stepping away before yelling, or accepting a boundary without retaliation.

Caregivers also need permission to require repair. It is not unkind to say, 'We need to talk about what happened,' or 'We need an apology,' or 'We need a plan before we pretend everything is fine.' Repair is one of the ways you protect children from emotional whiplash. Kids do not need perfect adults. They need adults who can return to safety after rupture.

Here is a practical tool that helps many families: a Repair Window. You choose a time when everyone is calm—maybe later that day, maybe the next day— when you agree to do a short repair conversation. If either person is escalated, you reschedule. This keeps repair from becoming another fight.

Repair also requires boundaries. Some ruptures are unsafe. Some involve violence, threats, or severe impairment. In those situations, repair may require professionals, supervision, or distance. Repair is not access at all costs. Repair is restoration where restoration is safe.

And for families of faith, repair is also discipleship. Scripture is full of confession, repentance, and restoration—not as shame, but as return. Repair says, 'We are not defined by our worst moment. We are defined by what we do next.' That is a legacy sentence for children to hear.

If you build repair into your family system, you will still have hard days—but you will have fewer lasting fractures. You will stop living in an endless cycle of rupture-without-return. And over time, trust can grow again—not because life is easy, but because your home is learning how to come back to peace.

Legacy Takeaway

Repair keeps rupture from becoming the family's identity. Short, honest repair conversations rebuild safety, restore dignity, and create a pathway back to trust.

Next Step

Choose one repair phrase you will use this week (e.g., 'I was wrong to yell. I'm sorry. I'm going to take a break sooner next time.'). Schedule one Repair Window after the next conflict.

Toolkit link:

Tool #28 — Repair Loop (4-Step Script + Repair Window Plan)

Closing Prayer

God, give us humility to repair quickly and courage to tell the truth without blame. Teach us to confess what is ours, to protect safety with wise boundaries, and to rebuild trust one faithful step at a time. Heal what has been damaged in our home, and let restoration become part of our legacy of stability. Amen.

Chapter 18
Crisis Wisdom: When to Escalate Care and How to Stay Grounded

No one wants to talk about crisis. Families would rather believe it won't happen again. Caregivers would rather not imagine the worst. And people who struggle would rather not face the vulnerability of needing higher-level care. [4]

But crisis is part of many mental illness stories, and preparedness is not pessimism. Preparedness is protection. It keeps the home from scrambling, it protects children from being exposed to chaos, and it gives the person who is struggling a clearer pathway to safety when their own clarity is low.

Here is the truth: in a crisis, the goal is not to prove a point. The goal is safety.

So this chapter is about crisis wisdom—how to recognize when care needs to escalate, how to act without panic, and how to stay grounded in the middle of high emotion.

First, let's clarify what we mean by "escalating care." Escalating care can mean several things depending on severity: calling a clinician for an urgent appointment, contacting a prescriber about medication concerns, using a crisis hotline or mobile crisis team, going to urgent care or the emergency department, involving law enforcement only when necessary for safety, or pursuing inpatient or intensive outpatient treatment.

Families often hesitate to escalate care because they fear conflict, stigma, cost, or relationship rupture. They worry the person will feel betrayed. They worry it will "make things worse." And sometimes they've had negative experiences with systems that felt harsh or confusing.

I understand those fears. But when safety is at risk, waiting is not love. Waiting is risk.

So how do you know when it's time to escalate? Here are common red flags families should take seriously: suicidal statements or plans, threats of harm to others, psychosis or severe delusions that impair reality testing, inability to sleep for several nights with escalating agitation, dangerous impulsivity, substance intoxication with unstable behavior, medical symptoms that could be medication-related, severe self-neglect, or repeated patterns where the person cannot keep themselves safe.

Notice that many of these are not about whether the person is being "difficult." They are about safety and reality.

Second, crisis wisdom includes a pre-decided plan.

A crisis plan is not a long document. It is a simple agreement that answers: Who calls whom? Where do we go? Who stays with children? What information do we bring? What are the key medications and diagnoses? What is the person's preferred hospital or facility? Who has permission to speak to clinicians? And what are the non-negotiables for safety?

A plan is particularly important because in crisis, the responsible caregiver's brain can go into overload. Decision-making becomes harder. Emotions get loud. Conflict can erupt between adults. Children can feel terrified. A plan reduces the chaos.

Third, crisis wisdom includes grounded leadership.

Grounded leadership does not mean you feel calm. It means you act calm. You slow your body down. You lower your voice. You speak in short sentences. You focus on the next right step. You do not argue with delusions. You do not try to "win" logic battles. You keep the person's dignity protected as much as possible while prioritizing safety.

This is also where co-regulation matters again. Your calm presence can keep the moment from becoming more explosive. Even if the person cannot receive your calm, your calm keeps you from being swept into panic.

Fourth, crisis wisdom protects children from adult crisis responsibility.

Children should not be the ones calling for help. They should not be the emotional support for the adult who is escalating. They should not be exposed to frightening scenes if it can be avoided. If there are kids in the home, the crisis plan must include: where the children go, who they are with, and what script they are told.

A child script can be simple: "Mom/Dad is not safe right now and needs help. You are safe. The adults are handling it. We are going to take care of you."

Fifth, crisis wisdom includes aftercare.

Many families breathe a sigh of relief after a crisis ends and then immediately return to "normal," hoping it won't happen again. But aftercare is where stability is rebuilt. Aftercare means follow-up appointments, medication review, therapy support, a calmer home rhythm, boundary adjustments, and often a renegotiated living plan. Aftercare also includes caregiver recovery—because crisis exposure is traumatic.

Let me name something else: it is possible to hold love and intervention together.

Families sometimes avoid escalation because they think it equals rejection. But escalation can be an act of love. It can communicate: "We will not pretend you're okay when you're not. We will help you get the level of care you need."

Now, a practical note: if you've never had to do this, it can feel intimidating. But you don't have to become an expert in crisis systems overnight. You can learn your local resources. You can store hotline numbers. You can ask your clinician what to do if symptoms escalate. You can build a simple emergency information sheet. These are small steps that make a big difference.

And if you are a person of faith, hear this: crisis does not mean God has failed you. Crisis means the brain is under strain, the nervous system is overwhelmed, and the system needs support. In those moments, prayer is not denial—it is strength. Prayer can keep you grounded and keep your tone soft while you take practical action.

So here is the core message: crisis readiness is part of building a legacy of stability. It protects children. It protects caregivers. It protects the person who is struggling. And it helps the family respond with wisdom instead of panic when the moment comes.

Legacy Takeaway

Preparedness is protection. A simple crisis plan and grounded leadership help families escalate care wisely when safety is at risk—without panic, shame, or unnecessary chaos.

Next Step

Create a one-page Crisis Readiness Sheet: emergency contacts, clinician/prescriber numbers, medications, diagnoses, preferred facility, child care plan, and your 'red flag' list for when to escalate care. Store it where you can access it quickly.

Toolkit link:

Tool #1 — Crisis Readiness Sheet + Tool #15 — Red Flag Decision Guide

Closing Prayer

God, give us wisdom and courage in moments of crisis. Help us act with steadiness, protect children, and pursue the care that is needed without shame. Guide our words, calm our bodies, and strengthen our home team to respond with clarity and love. When fear rises, anchor us in Your presence and lead us to the next right step. Amen.

Chapter 19
When Healing Doesn't Come This Side of Heaven: Enduring Love, Acceptance, and Ongoing Care

There is a chapter families rarely think they will need—until they do.

It is the chapter where you realize that while some mental illness can be managed and life can have seasons of calm, there are also stories where full recovery does not come. Not in the way you hoped. Not in the timeline you prayed for. Not in the tidy ending you wanted for the person you love—and for yourself.

If you are living in that reality, I want to speak to you with tenderness and truth. Because if we make "cure" the only acceptable definition of healing, many families will feel like they failed. And that is not only untrue—it is cruel.

In my years of ministry and pastoral counseling, I have prayed for miraculous breakthroughs, and I have also stood beside families who carried ongoing illness for decades. The tension is real: we believe God heals, and we also live in a world where suffering exists. We can hold hope for the miraculous and compassion for the chronic at the same time. Faith does not require denial. Faith requires presence.

Some families are living with medication-resistant illness. Some are living with chronic psychosis or severe mood instability. Some are living with cycles of relapse. Some are living with the gradual loss of cognition or reality testing. Some are living with the grief of watching someone they love drift into an alternate internal world. Those families carry an unseen heroism. They love through confusion. They show up when there is no applause. They build structure, repeat routines, and keep dignity intact even when the story feels unfair.

This is also where grief becomes complicated. You may grieve the loss of the person you remember while the person is still alive. You may grieve dreams you had for your family. You may grieve the version of "normal" you thought you would get. And you may grieve the way other people don't understand the weight you carry. That grief is real. It deserves compassion, not shame.

So what is healing if the illness remains?

Sometimes healing looks like peace within the storm rather than the storm's end. Sometimes it looks like a family learning to communicate without destroying each other. Sometimes it looks like a caregiver learning to rest without guilt. Sometimes it looks like children being protected and still growing into steady adults. Sometimes it looks like a person who still struggles but stays connected to care and community. Sometimes it looks like faith that remains anchored even when the mind does not fully recover.

I've seen this with my own eyes: cognition can falter and faith can endure. A person can be confused and still worship. A person can be unstable and still be loved by God. And a family can be weary and still be held by grace.

This is why I invite families to redefine wholeness. Wholeness is not the absence of struggle. Wholeness is living with dignity, support, and purpose in the story you actually have. Wholeness is a family system that no longer measures love by whether symptoms disappear. Wholeness is the presence of Christ in the middle of what you cannot fix.

This is also where acceptance becomes a holy word. Acceptance is not giving up. Acceptance is adjusting expectations in the light of reality while refusing to surrender dignity and love. Acceptance says, "We will stop fighting what is true, and we will build the structure that holds."

Acceptance also releases guilt. Mental illness is not a failure of faith or family. It is a medical, emotional, and spiritual battle that requires grace—for the person who is struggling and for the people who love them.

And acceptance brings us back to the Anchors of Support. When long-term illness is part of the story, families need the full team even more. The medical anchor helps monitor brain and body realities. The clinical anchor helps build skills and process grief and trauma. The community anchor helps reduce isolation and carry practical load. The home team protects children, boundaries, and daily rhythm. When one anchor tries to become all anchors, burnout follows. When the anchors work together, stability becomes possible—even when symptoms remain.

Let's talk about the spiritual ache that shows up here. Families sometimes feel betrayed by God when healing doesn't come the way they prayed. If you have felt that, you are not alone. Scripture is honest about suffering. The Psalms are full of questions. Jesus Himself wept. Faith is not pretending. Faith is bringing your real grief into the presence of a real God.

And we keep the eternal perspective without using it to bypass pain. We do not rush past grief with platitudes. We grieve, and we also remember the promise that broken minds and wounded hearts are not the final chapter. There will be a day when all is made whole. That hope is not denial. It is endurance.

So here is what I want you to carry from this chapter: if healing does not come in the way you hoped, you can still build a legacy of stability. Your legacy may look like faithfulness more than fireworks. It may look like structure, compassion, and shared support over the long haul. It may look like staying kind. It may look like protecting children. It may look like loving well in a complicated story.

And that, dear family, is not failure. That is discipleship. That is courageous love.

Legacy Takeaway

If cure becomes the only definition of healing, families carry unnecessary shame. Wholeness can also mean dignity, shared support, protected children, and enduring love—especially when the illness remains.

Next Step

Write your family's 'definition of wholeness' for this season in 3–5 sentences. Include what you will protect (safety, dignity, children, connection, purpose) and what support you will keep in place (Anchors). Share it with one trusted person on your support team.

Toolkit link:

Tool #30 — Redefining Wholeness Worksheet + Tool #31 — Grief and Endurance Support Plan

Closing Prayer

Lord, when healing does not come as we hoped, hold us steady in Your grace. Comfort the families who love through confusion, who stay when answers fade, and who trust You through pain they cannot fix. Give courage to caregivers, mercy to the weary, and hope to those who grieve. Teach us to see healing as You see it—in endurance, in compassion, and in the promise that one day, all will be made whole. Amen.

Appendix
The Legacy of Stability Toolkit

This toolkit is here so the chapters can stay clean and conversational while still giving you practical tools you can return to any time. Use this in whatever order fits your family. You don't have to do everything at once.

A simple way to use the toolkit is to start with two pages: Tool #1 (Crisis Readiness Sheet) and Tool #24 (Family Living Plan). Those two tools create immediate structure. Then add tools as you need them.

Remember: the goal is not perfection. The goal is a sustainable structure that protects safety, dignity, connection, and purpose—and can be renegotiated as life changes.

Tool #1 — Crisis Readiness Sheet (One Page)

- Purpose: A quick-reference page you can grab in a high-stress moment.

- Include: emergency contacts; clinician/prescriber numbers; current medications; diagnoses (if known); preferred facility; who has medical permission; child care plan; your escalation thresholds; and your calm scripts.

- Keep: one copy at home (safe place) and one digital copy you can access quickly.

Tool #2 — Anchors of Support Map

- Purpose: Identify the four supports that keep recovery standing.

- Write the names and contact info for: Medical Anchor, Clinical Anchor, Community Anchor, and Home Team roles.

- Note: If an anchor is missing, write your next best step to build it.

Tool #3 — Behavior Pattern Map (5 Categories)

- Purpose: Respond wisely without needing a diagnosis manual.

- Categories: Escalation, Shutdown, Avoidance, Impulsivity, Relational Disruption.

- Use: When tension rises, name the category first— then choose the matching response script.

Tool #4 — Matching Response Scripts (Quick Choices)

- Escalation: "We will talk when we're calm."

- Shutdown: "I'm here. We can talk when you're ready."

- Avoidance: "Let's choose one small step that fits capacity."

- Impulsivity: "We're using the guardrails we agreed on."

- Relational disruption: "We will protect children and repair with dignity."

Tool #5 — Capacity-Matched Expectations Guide

- Purpose: Keep expectations realistic without removing responsibility.

- Ask: What can this person do consistently in this season?

- Adjust: Increase slowly when stability grows; decrease during depletion seasons.

Tool #6 — Weekly Pattern Tracker (6 Weeks)

- Track weekly: sleep, mood, energy, functioning, conflict level, major triggers, treatment adherence.

- Bring to appointments: clearer data helps better care decisions.

Tool #7 — Early Warning Signs List

- Purpose: Catch shifts before crisis.

- Common signs: sleep drop, isolation, agitation, rapid speech, spending changes, substance use, skipping appointments, increased conflict.

- Add your family's personal signs and what helps early.

Tool #8 — De-escalation Plan (Home-Friendly)

- Purpose: Lower intensity without power struggle.

- Steps: lower voice; reduce stimulation; keep words short; offer two calm choices; take space; return later.

- Remember: safety first, resolution later.

Tool #9 — Co-Regulation Scripts

- "You're safe. I'm here."

- "Let's take a minute."

- "Breathe with me."

- "We can pause and come back."

Tool #10 — Active Listening Script

- Receive: stop rehearsing your response.

- Reflect: "What I'm hearing is…"

- Respond: empathy, curiosity, boundary, or pause.

- Add timing: "This matters. Let's talk when we're calm."

Tool #11 — Questions to Ask a Clinician/Prescriber

- "What are we treating first?"

- "What symptoms should we watch for?"

- "What are common medication side effects?"

- "What should we do if symptoms escalate?"

- "How will we measure progress?"

Tool #12 — Boundaries With Bridges Script

- Boundary: "I'm willing to talk, but not while we are yelling."

- Bridge: "I want to understand you. Let's talk when we're calm."

- Rule: set fewer boundaries, but keep them.

Tool #13 — The 'Yucky Gut' Boundary Check

- When you feel irritated/discombobulated, ask: What limit is being crossed?

- Is this a capacity issue, access issue, or role drift issue?

- Choose: clarify the boundary, rotate the role, or add support.

Tool #14 — Dignity Language Swap List

- Swap character attacks for observations.

- Use: "I'm noticing…" "I hear you…" "This feels heavy…"

- Avoid: "You always…" "You're crazy…" "You ruin everything…"

Tool #15 — Red Flag Decision Guide

- Escalate care when: suicidal threats/plan, harm threats, severe psychosis, dangerous impulsivity, severe insomnia with agitation, intoxication with instability, medical concerns.

- When in doubt: consult clinician/prescriber or crisis resources.

Tool #16 — Child Safety Plan (Simple)

- Where do children go during adult escalation?

- Who is the safe adult contact?

- What is the child script?

- How do we keep kids out of adult messengers/triangulation?

Tool #17 — Aftercare Checklist (Post-Crisis)

- Follow-up appointments scheduled

- Medication review completed

- Living plan updated

- Caregiver rest scheduled

- Child debrief (age-appropriate) completed

- Support team notified (as needed)

Tool #18 — Caregiver Capacity Check

- List: what I'm carrying; what can be shared; what can be reduced.

- Name: one support to add; one boundary to clarify; one rest practice to protect.

- Repeat monthly or after crisis seasons.

Tool #19 — Permission Statements (For Guilt)

- "I am allowed to rest."

- "I am allowed to need help."

- "I am allowed to renegotiate what I can carry."

- "I can love without unlimited access."

Tool #20 — Home Team Role List

- Finance, logistics, child care, meal rhythm, appointment coordination, crisis caller, community connector, boundary keeper, repair leader.

- Choose roles based on capacity and skill—not fairness pressure.

Tool #21 — Matching Response Scripts (Expanded)

- Write your family's preferred scripts for each pattern category.

- Keep it short, kind, repeatable.

- Post it where adults can see it.

Tool #22 — Repair Phrases (Short + True)

- "I was sharp. I'm sorry."

- "I raised my voice. That wasn't okay."

- "I got defensive. I want to try again."

- "I care about you, and I want us to be okay."

Tool #23 — Role Rotation Map

- Which role is too heavy right now?

- Who can rotate in—family, friend, community, professional?

- When will we review the rotation (date)?

Tool #24 — Family Living Plan (One Page)

- (1) What we're building (main thing)

- (2) Who does what (Anchors + roles)

- (3) Non-negotiables (safety/dignity)

- (4) Response pathway when things get hard

- Review monthly for three months, then quarterly.

Tool #25 — Non-Negotiables Builder

- Start with child safety and basic dignity.

- Examples: no threats, no violence, no adult conflict in front of kids, no substance use in the home, no intimidation, no using kids as messengers.

- Write consequences you can actually follow through on.

Tool #26 — Emotional Regression Quick Guide (Do's/Don'ts)

- Do: stay calm, validate feelings, offer simple choices, protect dignity, use grounding.

- Don't: shame, flood with logic, touch without permission, argue while dysregulated.

- After: gently ask what felt triggering.

Tool #27 — Connection Menu (Small + Sustainable)

- 10-minute check-in, shared meal, short walk, scheduled call, quiet presence, prayer together, supportive text.

- Choose what fits capacity and safety.

Tool #28 — Purpose Builder (Capacity-Matched Roles)

- Pick one role the person can carry consistently (small and faithful).

- Examples: pet care, one task, art/writing, group attendance, volunteering small.

- Review and adjust as capacity changes.

Tool #29 — Child-Safe Talking Points

- "Mom/Dad is not well right now, and adults are helping."

- "You are safe."

- "This is not your fault."

- "You can love your parent and still have boundaries."

Tool #30 — Redefining Wholeness Worksheet

- Write 3–5 sentences: what wholeness means in this season.

- Include: what you will protect and what supports you will keep.

- Share with a trusted support person.

Tool #31 — Grief and Endurance Support Plan

- Name your grief (losses, changes, ongoing realities).

- Name your supports (people, counseling, respite, faith community).

- Name your endurance practices (sleep, rhythm, prayer, boundaries, joy).

A Final Note

If you only do two things this month, do these: (1) build your Anchors of Support map, and (2) write your one-page Family Living Plan. Those two steps alone can lower chaos and raise hope.

Keep going. Small, steady actions build a legacy.

Endnotes

Citation system: Tier 1 uses bracketed reference numbers in the text (e.g., [4]). Tier 2 provides full APA-style source details in the Bibliography/Recommended Reading section below.

Tier 1 — Foundational Sources

1. Amen, D. G. (2015). Change your brain, change your life (Rev. ed.). Harmony Books.

2. van der Kolk, B. A. (2014). The body keeps the score: Brain, mind, and body in the healing of trauma. Viking.

3. Perry, B. D., & Szalavitz, M. (2017). The boy who was raised as a dog (Rev. ed.). Basic Books.

4. Siegel, D. J. (2012). The developing mind: How relationships and the brain interact to shape who we are (2nd ed.). Guilford Press.

Tier 2 — Supporting Sources

5. Cloud, H., & Townsend, J. (1992). Boundaries: When to say yes, how to say no to take control of your life. Zondervan.

Recommended Reading and Resources

This book is designed to support—not replace—professional medical and mental health care. If you need immediate help, contact local emergency services or a trusted crisis resource in your area.

Suggested categories to explore with your care team:

- Family psychoeducation and caregiver support

- Trauma-informed care and nervous system regulation

- Parenting support for families impacted by mental illness

- Faith-community mental health initiatives and referral networks

About the Author

Cindy H. Carr, D.Min., MACL, has spent her vocational life walking alongside people in the slow, often unseen work of formation and change. Her career has been intentionally bi-vocational, shaped by years of pastoring, business leadership, and pastoral counseling—always with a focus on helping people live with greater clarity, dignity, and wholeness.

She earned a Master of Arts in Church Leadership from Eastern Mennonite Seminary and completed her doctoral work at Liberty University. Over the years, she served multiple churches in Virginia's Shenandoah Valley in a variety of pastoral and leadership capacities.

In this season of life, Cindy's work has shifted from direct leadership into writing and education. Through her books, she helps readers implement formation-based principles she has taught throughout her career—practices centered on identity, connection, return, and steady growth without shame.

Learn more about Cindy and her work at
CindyHCarr.com

www.ingramcontent.com/pod-product-compliance
Lightning Source LLC
Chambersburg PA
CBHW071224240726
48654CB00009B/909